I0423902

Low Carb High

Fat Diet

The all in one Banting guide to losing weight and staying healthy

ROSE POTTER

©2016

INTRODUCTION

Most individuals in the world are looking to lose weight and to get fit. This is a difficult goal especially in current times, as obesity has become an epidemic over the past decade. Research has shown that 65% of the people in the world are living in countries where obesity is killing more people than many other health related problems. This comes despite the advances of modern medicine and research, and easy access to diet and health information and access to gyms and exercise classes.

I recommend researching the different diets out there before deciding on the one that best one for you. However, you may find that many diets are preaching the wrong things. After considering all the research I have done on this topic, I am beginning to realise that our thinking regarding dieting over the past decade may be flawed!

People believe that they should avoid fat at all costs when dieting. I believe that this pattern of thinking is about to change. In fact, it is sugar that we should be avoiding like the plague. A low-carb diet restricts sugary foods, and starches like pasta and bread. This diet means you eat fewer carbohydrates and instead eat a higher proportion of fat. This is often called a low-carb, high fat (LCHF) diet. Many high-quality scientific studies show that a low-carb diet makes it easier both to lose weight and to control your blood sugar, and that is just the beginning. Carbohydrates are believed to be the main sources of weight gain and diabetes, and the intake of these should always be in moderation. This book guides you on how to follow a Low-Carb, High Fat diet so as to achieve weight loss and many other health benefits associated with this diet.

Enjoy reading!

Table of Contents

Chapter 1- Why Low-Carb Diet?

A low-carb diet means that you eat fewer carbohydrates and higher fat proportion. This is what is usually referred to as low-carb, high fat diet (LCHF). The most important thing with such a diet is that you reduce your intake for starches and sugar. Instead of relying on such foods, there are other delicious foods that you can eat, feel satisfied and reduce weight. Research has shown that with a low-carb diet, one can find it easy to lose weight and control their blood sugar.

With a low-carb diet, one can experience an effortless weight loss plan. This type of diet is also good for reversing the type 2 diabetes and some other health benefits. With a low-carb diet, you are not expected to count calories, nor are you expected to take pills or undergo a surgery. All you have to do is to eat real food. Instead of eating starches such as bread or pasta, or sugary foods, you eat real foods such as natural fats, vegetables and proteins, which are delicious.

How the Diet works

During the early days, human beings were hunters and gatherers, meaning that they did not rely on too many carbohydrates. They relied on natural foods by hunting, fishing and gathering anything which was edible to them. Foods such as rice, pasta and bread contain pure starch, but the early foods did not have these. These starchy foods came to existence once agriculture was developed. Our genes have not fully adapted to such foods.

With industrial revolution, which began in the past 100-200 years, factories began to manufacture huge amounts of white flour and pure sugar. Our bodies have not had enough time to adapt to such processed foods.

The western world began to fear fats in the 80s, and this led to manufacture of low-fat products. However, after eating low fats, one has to eat more carbohydrates so as to feel satiated. As a result, the epidemics of diabetes and obesity began. However, the today's world has realized that fearing real food having natural fats is the greatest mistake we have made.

Effects of Sugar and Starch

All carbohydrates which the body can digest are broken down to get simple sugars once they reach the intestines. The resulting sugar is absorbed into our bloodstream, which causes an increase in blood glucose levels. The body in turn reacts to this by increasing the production of insulin, which is a hormone for fat storage.

The pancreas is responsible for production of insulin. When this is released in large amounts, it will prevent the body from burning fat, and facilitate the storage of nutrients in the fat cells. If this goes on for some time, the blood will end up lacking some nutrients, and you will hunger and crave for a sweet food. At this point, most people will eat. The process will begin again, and one experiences weight gain.

On the other hand, if you take a low-carb diet, you achieve a stable and lower blood glucose level, and the level of insulin gets lower. The fat stores begin to release fats, which is then burned. This causes the body to lose fat, and especially the one stored in the belly, and one experiences weight lose.

Lose Weight without Feeling Hunger

With LCHF diet, the body will make use of the fats stored in the reserves, as the insulin levels will not be high enough to block the release of the fats. This explains why one feels satiety for long after eating fats than carbohydrates.

With such a diet, you will not need to count or weight your food. You just have to forget the calories and trust your hunger and satiety feelings.

Chapter 2- What you should Eat

You are now asking yourself what are the kinds of foods that you should eat? For example, what can you eat for breakfast? And for what should you substitute the bread or pasta? Let us give you list of the low-carb foods that you should eat.

LOW-CARB VEGETABLES

1. Cauliflower- a cup of cauliflower has 5 grams of carbs. After cooking these, they have a unique texture which we can use as a substitute for mashed potatoes, creamy soups, pizza crust, mac and cheese. You can also pulverize a whole head of cauliflower in food processor and then use it as a substitute for rice or couscous. Cauliflower is also rich in antioxidants.

2. Zucchini- this is a good vegetable for reducing the amount of carbs that your diet has. Use a spiralizer or serrated vegetable peeler to cut this into noodle-looking strands and use it as a substitute for spaghetti which is dense in carbohydrates.

   One can use grated zucchinis for hash browns in potato lieu or add them to pancake batter.

To get a low-carb snack, just slice off the ends of zucchini and then use a mandolin or vegetable peeler to make wide, long strips. Place some arugula or smoked salmon at the end of each of your zucchini ribbon and then roll up.

3. Swiss Chard- dark, nutrient-dense, leafy greens should be added to grocery cart, and this is also the case with Swiss chard. You can choose to sauté or steam the leaves, or use them when whole and uncooked as a substitute for carb-heavy tortillas when you are making wraps or tacos.

4. Celery- water makes 95% of celery, which explains why it is low in carbohydrates. Slice and add it to salad, or smear nut butter on it to make a snack.

5. Mushrooms- each cup of mushrooms provides 2 grams of carbs. Although they are low in carbs, they are very rich in umami flavor. The large and meaty mushroom cups can be used as an alternative to hamburger buns, or for replacing pizza crust. You just have to lay it on the pizza toppings.

6. Cherry Tomatoes- a cup of these provides 6 grams of carbs. Their flavor is better than that of the large tomatoes. They have few carbohydrates, making them a good source of low-carb diet. To get a sweet snack, just pop these into your mouth, or toss using oil and bake in an oven at 400 degrees F.

7. Spaghetti Squash- a cup of these provides 7 grams of carbohydrates. After cooking these, their flesh will pull apart to get noodle-like, nutty-tasting strands with no carbohydrate

deluge. Take a spaghetti squash and slice it into half lengthwise, then scoop the seeds out, and add the squash halves into a microwave dish. Use a paper towel to cover the squash loosely and microwave it for 8-12 minutes. You can also use a parchment paper to cover the squash. Allow the squash to stand for about 5 minutes, and then scrape the squash flesh out using a fork. Top it with meat sauce of choice.

LOW-CARB FRUITS

1. Avocado- a ½ piece of avocado provides 8 grams of carbs. Avocado is a fruit, and it has no sugar. The good news is that 75% of the carbs found in avocado are made up of non-digestible fiber.

2. Apricots- apricots are known for their low-sugar content, meaning that they are part of low-carb diet. You can enjoy this fruit as a snack, or slice it and add to yoghurt, salad or oatmeal for some natural sweetness.

3. Strawberries- a cup of strawberries provides 11 grams of carbs. They are the berry fruits with the lowest sugar levels.

4. Red Grapefruit- ½ piece of this provides 9 grams of carbs. It provides 20% less sugar

compared to the one provided by orange.

Although it is sour, do not coat it with sugar.

LOW-CARB FISH AND MEATS

1. Catfish- each 3 ounces of catfish provide 0 grams of carbs. It has more flavor than tilapia, and it helps you provide your body with pure proteins. The American farmed one is the best.

2. Chicken drumsticks- these provide 0 grams of carbs for per 3 ounces. They are rich in flavor and less likely to dry when you are cooking them. When cooking, leave the skin on so as to get more flavor, but if you don't like the calories in it, just strip it before you can eat.

3. Canned pink salmon- this provides 0 grams of carbs per ½ can. The canned one is a great source of carb-free diet. Pink salmon is the best and economical option as it is low in toxins that what you can find in canned tuna. This fish is

also rich in omega-3 fatty acids which are of great benefit to our health.

4. Pork Tenderloin- this provides 0 grams of carb per 3 ounces. It is cheap and has a rich flavor when not overcooked compared to beef. We recommend that you go for the unseasoned pork tenderloin as this is free of salt and other ingredients which may not be healthy to you.

5. Ground Turkey- this provides 0 grams of carbs per 3 ounces. Go for the inexpensive one and you will get a carb-free protein. You can use this for meat sauces and burgers.

6. Roast beef- this provides 0 grams of carbs per 2 ounces. It has no sugars and this makes it one of the best source low-carb diets. Just wrap some roast beef slices and some roasted red pepper, Dijon mustard smear and some

avocado or cheese in collard leaves or large Swiss chard.

7. Top Sirloin Steak- this provides 0 grams of carbs per 3 ounces. It provides you with a carb-free protein diet at a low cost. You can make use of marinades, and this will help in tenderizing your meat. Splurge for steak obtained from cattle fed on grass so as to boost the nutritional value.

8. Bison- this provides 0 grams of carbs per each 3 ounces, meaning that it provides you with a carb-free diet. You can easily find these from nearest butcher counters as most people have now turned to the paleo lifestyle, looking for alternatives to beef.

LOW-CARB DAIRY

1. Butter- each tablespoon of butter provides 0 grams of carbs. You can blend butter with steamed cauliflower some pinches of salt and fresh thyme. You can then add these to some mashed potatoes for a great taste. Avoid using substitutes of butter such as such as margarine as these are rich in cholesterol and this can increase your risk of cardiovascular disease.

2. Gruyere Cheese- each ounce of this provides 0 grams of carbs. Use it as a substitute for mundane cheese slices and you will get a great nutty taste. It also exhibits a good melting habit, and this makes it a good source of excitement to low-carb pizzas and broccoli.

3. Eggs- 2 large eggs provide 1 gram of carbs. Both the chicken and the egg will provide with

a protein-rich diet with no much carbohydrates. Research has also shown that eggs are rich in good protein than any whole food you can find. These are also rich in antioxidants and they can help your body fight the radicals which can damage your cells.

4. Plain Greek Yoghurt- each cup of this provides 9 grams of carbs. It is rich in proteins, as a cup of this will provide 23 grams of proteins. It is also good for your muscles, and this is why you can't afford to avoid this. To get a carb-free or low-carb diet, go for the plain greek yoghurt as these has not been sweetened with sugar.

5. Cottage Cheese- each cup of cottage cheese provides 6 grams of carbs and 28 grams of proteins. This is why it is common for individuals in need of building their body. Some brands can be rich in sodium, so ensure

that you compare the available brands. You can take it as a snack in the evening to ensure that the muscle making process continues as you snooze away.

6. Goat Milk- each cup of goat milk provides 11 grams of carbs. It has less carbs compared to the cow milk and it is digested easily. Research has also shown that goat milk has other nutrients such as the omega-3 fatty acids which are of health benefits to our bodies.

LOW-CARB PLANT PROTEINS

1. Tofu- each 3 ounces of tofu provides us with 3 grams of carbs. However, it is only taken by vegetarians. It can provide you with a low-carb protein diet. When alone, you can't enjoy its taste, but after adding it to foods such as sauces, you will enjoy the taste. Stir-fry it as a cheap protein, or slap it on grill.

2. Canned Pinto Beans- ½ cup of pinto beans provides 18 grams of carbs. They provide the lowest number of carbs among the canned beans, but they are rich in plant proteins, as each serving provides 12 grams of proteins. Add these to scrambled eggs and salads to boost the level of protein in these. They are rich I n fiber, and these are good in preventing

spiking of the blood sugar caused by intake of a carbohydrate-rich meal.

3. Tempeh- each 3 ounces of tempeh provides 9 grams of carbs. It is made from fermented soybeans, and this explains why it is an excellent source of proteins. It has a nutty, earthy and smoky flavor. Crumble it and add to stir-fry, chilli, soups, tacos, pasta sauce and casseroles. Since it is a fermented product, tempeh is believed to be rich in ultra-healthy probiotics.

4. Pumpkin Seeds- each ounce of pumpkin seeds provides 5 grams of carbs. They are good source of protein, as each serving provides 7 grams of whole-food proteins. Their carbohydrates are sugar-free, and this makes them a good way for boosting the level of

proteins in oatmeal, salads, cottage cheese or yoghurt.

LOW-CARB SNACKS

1. String Cheese- 3 grams of string cheese provide 0 grams of carbs. They are good for both children and adults. The prepackaged string cheese is a great source of low-carb snacks. String cheese is also rich in dairy-proteins, and these are good for boosting the strength of your muscles. It is also rich in calcium, and this is good for healthy and string bones.

2. Walnuts- each ounce of walnuts provides 4 grams of carbs. They provide you with a rich protein diet free of carbs, and they are rich in omega-3 fatty acids which are good for your health. Ensure that you take salt-free ones as this will help you check the amount of sodium that you take. It will also provide your body

with copper, which is a good nutrient for boosting the amount of energy in your body.

3. Kale Chips- each ounce of kale chips provides 8-12 grams of carbs. The crispy kale chips have a nice taste, and they are very dense in nutrients. When comapted to the potato-based chips, kale chips will provide you with 30% less carbohydrates, and this is good for your health. Besides having lo carbs, kale chips are rich in vitamin C, vitamin A and vitamin K.

LOW-CARB FLOUR/GRAINS

1. Almond flour- ¼ cup of almond flour provides 6 grams of carbs. Finely ground almonds are used for making almond flour, making them for use in baked foods such as pancakes, and this can give you that six-pack you have been yearning for.

2. Amaranth- each ½ cup of amaranth provides 23 grams of carbs. Amaranths are a type of grains with lower amounts of carbohydrates compared to the other types of grains. They are also rich in the essential amino acids just like the quinoa and these are good for building your body muscles. Just cook the in water, and they will release the starch in them. Use them as a substitute for oats when preparing your breakfast porridge. They also supply your body

with significant amounts of manganese, which is good for digestion of copper.

3. Shirataki Noodles- each 3 ounce of these noodles provides you with 0 grams of carbs. They are made from the root of konjac yam plant and majority of its parts are made up of indigestible fiber which can give you a carb-free diet. They usually add a good flavor to sauces. Drain and then rinse them very well, and then blanch the in some boiling water. It is also good for individuals with Type 2 diabetes as it helps in regulating the level of blood sugar and improves the level of cholesterol in our body.

LOW-CARB DRINKS

1. Unsweetened Iced Tea- this is made up of water and brewed tea, providing the body with 0 grams of carbs per cup. It is good in quenching thirst, and it can help in losing your weight. Go for the one made of green tea and combine it with some physical exercise. This will help you boost fat metabolism in your body and you will shed some pounds.

2. Maple Water- each cup of this provides 3 grams of carbs. We make this from maple tree, and it gives us half the amount of sugar we get from coconut water, Each sip of this will give a similar taste to the one you get from your morning flapjacks. Besides having lows carbs, it will provide your body with manganese which is good for healthy bones.

3. Unsweetened Almond Milk- each cup of this has only 2 grams of carbohydrates. It is a drink based on nuts, and good for adding to cereals or protein cereals, and it will not change the amount of carbs in the diet. Most of the available non-dairy beverages are sweetened with sugars, so ensure that you go for the ones labeled "unsweetened" so as to avoid the sugars which increase the amount of carbs in these. Other than having low carbs, it will also boost the level of vitamin E in your body which is good for a healthy living.

4. Tomato Juice- each cup of tomato juice provides 10 grams of carbohydrates. Research has shown that the tomato juice provides the body with ½ less the amount of sugars we get from orange juice. Diets are important as they protect us against the risk of water detention.

Also, it will be good for you to ensure that you rely on juice which is 100% vegetable, but avoid the ones sweetened with sugar.

Chapter 3- Healthy Low-Carb Recipes

Breakfast

Vegetables and Eggs

Ingredients:

- Coconut oil

- Spinach

- Frozen Vegetable Mix (cauliflower, carrots, green beans, broccoli)

- Spices

Directions:

1. Add the coconut oil into a frying pan and begin to heat.

2. Add in vegetables, followed by 3-4 eggs.

3. Add in the spices. If you have a spice mix, the better, but you can also use pepper and salt.

4. If you have spinach, add them in.

5. Stir fry the mixture until ready.

Egg and Sausage Bites

Ingredients:

- 1 bunch of dark greens, like kale, beet greens, Swiss chard or spinach
- 1-2 cups of uncooked, crumbled sausage
- 8-10 eggs
- a bunch of parsley/fresh herb

Directions:

1. Begin by preheating the oven up to 375 F.

2. Slice the greens so as to get thin stripes, Saute in butter or oil over some medium heat for some minutes. Add in the crumbled sausage.

3. Saute more until the sausage gets cooked, and turn the heat off.

4. Whist your eggs, add the kale, sausage and parsley and stir.

5. Pour the above into a greased pan. Bake for about 20-25 minutes.

6. Cool and then cut into squares.

Cowboy Breakfast Skillet

Ingredients:

- 1 lb of breakfast sausage
- 1 diced avocado
- 2 diced medium sweet potatoes
- 5 eggs
- handful cilantro
- hot sauce
- s & p
- raw cheese (optional)

Directions:

1. Begin by preheating the oven until it reaches 400°F.

2. In a skillet over medium heat, crumble the sausage until it turns brown.

3. Remove the sausage using a slotted spoon and hang it while cooking sweet potatoes. Reserve as much grease as you can.

4. Toast sweet potatoes into sausage grease and then allow them to get cooked and greased.

5. Take the pan and then add your sausage back into it.

6. Make some wells in the well, one for each of your eggs. Crack the eggs into these wells.

7. Put the skillet in your oven. Bake this for about 5 minutes so that the eggs can be set.

8. Turn your oven to broil, then heat the top part of the eggs for some minutes, but do not let the yolk to be cooked too much, but if you do not like runny yolks, cook much.

9. Remove your pan from oven, douse the whole of the thin g with avocado, hot sauce and cilantro.

10. To serve, use a large spoon to scoop out an egg alongside its goodies.

Broccoli and Cheese Egg Omelets

Ingredients:

- fresh pepper and salt
- 4 cups of broccoli florets
- 1 cup of egg whites
- 4 whole eggs (large)
- 1/4 cup of shredded cheddar (Sargento)
- 1 tsp of olive oil

- 1/4 cup of cheese such as pecorino romano (good grated)
- cooking spray

Directions:

1. Begin by preheating the oven up to 350°.
2. Use little water to steam the broccoli for 6-7 minutes.
3. Once the broccoli gets cooked, crumble it into smaller pieces and then add in some olive oil, pepper and salt. Mix these well.
4. Take a cooking spray and use it to spray a nonstick tin. Spray your broccoli mixture into the 9 tins evenly.
5. Take a medium bowl and then beat the eggs, egg whites, salt, pepper and grated cheese into it. Pour this into the greased tins over the broccoli until they are over ¾ full.

6. Top this with some grated cheddar and then bake in an oven until they are cooked, which should take about 20 minutes.

7. Serve immediately. In case of any leftovers, wrap them in a plastic wrap and place in a refrigerator.

Tex-Mex Scramble

Ingredients:

- 5 eggs
- 2 Tbsp of Pace Salsa
- 2 Tbsp water
- 1/8 cup red onion (chopped)
- 2 diced cherry tomatoes
- 1/8 cup green pepper (chopped)
- 1/2 cup thawed and drained frozen spinach
- 1 slice of pepper jack cheese

- 5 chopped jalapeno pepper slices

Directions:

1. Add canola oil to the skillet and begin to heat over medium heat.

2. Mix water, eggs, onion, pepper, tomatoes, jalapenos and spinach together. Pour them into oiled pan placed over medium heat and heat until you get the desired consistency from the eggs.

3. Once the eggs are ready for removal, turn off the heat and then add in the pepper jack cheese at the top. Use a pan, a lid or a plate to cover this and then allow it to sit for about 5 minutes.

4. Add in some 2 Tbsp salsa and then serve it immediately.

Savory Cheese Chive Waffles

Ingredients:

- 1 cup raw, processed cauliflower

- 1/3 cup of Parmesan cheese (shredded)

- 1 tsp of garlic powder

- 1 cup of mozzarella shredded cheese (processed)

- 1 tsp of onion powder

- 1/2 of tsp pepper

- 1 Tbsp chives

- 2 eggs

- sun-dried tomatoes (optional)

- fresh parsley (optional)

Directions:

1. Heat the waffle maker up to when it becomes ready.

2. Add some scant ¼ cups readily filled with butter to the griddle. Set your timer for 4-6

minutes and peek after minute 4. In case the maker sticks, give it some more time to cook.

3. Once cooked, remove it and then cool it in a plate. Refrigerate the remaining one.

Breads

Oopsie Rolls

Ingredients:

- Nonstick cooking spray
- ⅛ teaspoon salt
- ⅛ teaspoon of tartar cream
- 3 large eggs
- 3 ounces of full-fat cream cheese (cubed, cold)

Directions:

1. Begin by preheating the oven until it reaches 300 degree F. Line a parchment paper on a cookie sheet and then spray it with non-stick spray.

2. Separate your eggs, ensuring that no yolks get into the whites and then place the whites in a non-greasy, clean bowl.

3. Use a non-greasy, clean electric whisk to whip your egg whites and tartar cream until it becomes stiff.

4. Whisk the cream cheese, yolks and salt in a separate bowl until they become smooth.

5. Use a spatula to fold your egg whites your cream cheese mixture, doing it in batches. Just place the egg whites on the yolk mixture, then fold your yolk mixture from the egg whites, while rotating the bowl until the mixture becomes well incorporated. Te folding technique should be used because we are in need of keeping the air bubble intact in our egg whites.

6. Take a baking sheet and then spoon the mixture into it, up to 6 spoons. Press this gently with a spatula so as to flatten it.

7. Bake until it becomes golden brown, or for about 30-40 minutes.

8. Cool it for a number of minutes , then transfer it into a wire rack for further cooling. Store the leftovers in a refrigerator for some days.

Cheesy Garlic Bread

Ingredients:

- 1/2 tsp. of guar gum or xanthan
- 1 1/4 C of almond flour
- 3 egg whites
- 2 T of olive oil (you can also use avocado oil)
- 1 T of coconut flour
- 1/4 C of warm water
- 1 tsp. of coconut sugar (or molasses or honey)
- 1/2 C of shredded mozzarella cheese
- 1 tsp. of live yeast granules
- 1/4 tsp. salt

- 1/4 tsp. of garlic powder

- 2 tsp. of baking powder

Topping:

- 1 C of shredded mozzarella cheese

- 1/4 tsp. of garlic powder

- 2 T melted butter

- 1/2 tsp. of Italian seasoning

- 1/4 tsp. salt

Directions:

1. Begin by preheating the oven until it reaches 400 degrees.

2. Combine the salt, coconut flour, almond milk, garlic powder, xanthan gum and baking powder in a large bowl. Stir well until combined.

3. Take a small bowl o cup and combine warm water and sugar in it. Add in the yeast and then set aside for some minutes.

4. Add the yeast-water mixture and olive oil into your flour mixture and use a rubber spatula to stir well. Add the beaten eggs and go on with mixing.

5. Add 1/2 C mozzarella shreds, use your spatula to mix well until you get a nice dough. The cheese should also be mixed well.

6. Take a square pan and grease it well. Take a cake pan and add your batter into it. Make a square or rectangle from the dough.

7. Bake this for about 15-17 minutes, or until the crust sides turn into golden brown. Remove from heat and then top.

8. Take a tiny bowl and then combine the garlic powder, butter and salt. Mix these well, and then brush them over the garlic bread base.

9. Use some shredded mozzarella cheese to top the bread, then use Italian seasoning for spraying.

10. Bake for 10 minutes at 400 degrees until the cheese melts. During the last 3 minutes, turn on the broiler so that the cheese can become brown.

11. Remove it from oven, and allow the bread to sit for about 5-10 minutes and then serve.

Low Carb Bread

Ingredients:

- 1½ cups of almond flour
- ¼ cup of flaxseed meal
- ¼ tspn salt

- 1 tspn sweetener

- 1½ tspn of baking soda

- 5 eggs

- ¼ cup of coconut oil

- 2 tblspn of coconut flour

- 1 tblspn of apple cider vinegar

Directions:

1. Begin by preheating the oven until it reaches 180C/350F. Grease your loaf pan.

2. Place the coconut flour, almond flour, salt, baking soda and flax in your food processor.

3. Pulse together the ingredients.

4. Add in the oil, eggs and vinegar and then pulse.

5. Take the loaf pan and pour the batter into it.

6. Poor for 30 minutes at 350 degrees.

7. Cool and then serve.

Low-Carb Lunches

Chicken Wings with Salsa and Greens

Ingredients:

- Chicken Wings
- Spices
- Some Greens
- Salsa

Directions:

1. Put the spice on the chicken wings. In my case, I have used chicken spice mix.

2. Place in an oven, and heat for about 40 minutes at 180-200°C.

3. Grill until the wings become crunchy and brown.

4. Serve with some salsa and vegetables.

Bacon and Eggs

Ingredients:

- Bacon
- Eggs

Directions:

1. Add your bacon to a pan and then fry until ready.
2. Put it on a plate, and then fry 3-4 eggs in bacon fat.
3. In case you need to add in some flavor to the eggs, add some bit of sea salt, onion powder and garlic powder on these as they fry.

Ground Beef with Bell Peppers (Sliced)

Ingredients:

- Coconut Oil
- Onions

- Ground Beef

- Spinach

- Spices

- Bell Pepper

Directions:

1. Cut your onion into small slices.

2. Add some coconut oil into a pan and then begin to heat.

3. Add the cut onion into the pan and then stir for about 1 minute.

4. Add in the ground beef.

5. Add in some spices. You can use spice mix, but pepper and salt will also work well.

6. Add in spinach.

7. If you are in need of getting more flavor, add in chilli powder and black pepper.

8. Stir fry these until they are ready, serve with some sliced bell pepper.

Cheeseburgers

Ingredients:

- Butter
- Hamburgers
- Cheddar Cheese
- Cream Cheese
- Salsa
- Spices
- Spinach

Directions:

1. Add some butter into a pan and then begin to heat.
2. Add spices and burgers.
3. Flip until they are almost ready.
4. Add cream cheese and some slices of cheddar to the top.

5. Turn the heat down and then cover with a lid for the cheese to melt.

6. Serve using some spinach. If you need, pour some fat from the pan into your spinach.

7. If you need to make these tastier, just pour some salsa on top.

Fried Chicken Breasts

Ingredients:

- Butter
- Chicken Breast
- Salt
- Pepper
- Garlic Powder
- Curry and Vegetables

Directions:

1. Cut the chicken breasts to get small pieces.

2. Add some butter to a pan and then begin to heat.

3. Add in the chicken pieces.

4. Add pepper, garlic powder, salt and curry.

5. Stir fry this until the chicken becomes brown and in a crunchy texture.

6. Serve this with some greens.

Moroccan Meatballs

Ingredients:

MeatBalls

- 1/2 cup fresh, minced parsley leaves
- 1/4 teaspoon of ground black pepper
- 2 teaspoons of ground cumin
- 1 teaspoon salt
- 1 tablespoon paprika
- 2 pounds of ground lamb

Sauce

- 1 tablespoon of coconut oil
- 2 medium diced onions
- 2 minced garlic cloves
- 2 teaspoons paprika
- 2 teaspoons of ground cumin
- 1 teaspoon salt
- 1/4 teaspoon of ground black pepper
- 2 medium diced tomatoes (about 2 cups)
- 1 1/2 cups water
- 2/3 cup of tomato paste
- 1/2 cup fresh, minced parsley leaves (about 2 tablespoons)
- garnish: 1/4 cup chopped, roasted pistachios

Directions:

1. Use a fork to combine parsley, cumin, paprika, salt, and pepper in a large bowl. Take a bowl

and using your hands, crumble the lamb into it. Knead these until you have all your ingredients incorporated.

2. Use water to moisten your hands, shake to remove excess one. Measure a tablespoon of lamb and then roll it into a ball in between your palms. Take a baking sheet and line the meatballs on it until time for putting them in a sauce comes.

3. Take a large, deep pot or skillet and then heat some oil in it. Add in the onion and sauté for about 5 minutes. Add in the salt, garlic, cumin, paprika, and pepper and then stir for about 30 seconds.

4. Add in some tomato paste and stir fry these for about 1 minute. Add in chopped tomatoes, water, and parsley and then stir well until well combined.

5. Boil the sauce, then add the meatballs to a skillet gently, cover them and then bring the heat to a simmer. Take 40 minutes to cook when covered. Remove the cover, then heat for further 20 minutes, and the sauce will become thick. Sprinkle the servings with some teaspoons of pistachios. You can then serve over cauliflower rice roasted over oven.

Low-Carb Salads

Bacon, Avocado, Egg and Tomato Salad

Ingredients:

- 1 ripe avocado (cut into chunks)
- 1 medium-sized tomato (cut into chunks)
- 2 boiled eggs (cut into chunks)
- 2-4 pieces of cooked bacon, crumbled
- Salt and pepper
- Juice from one lemon wedge

Directions:

Mix all of your ingredients, but do not stir too much.

BLT CHICKEN SALAD

Ingredients:

- 1 boneless, grilled chicken breast

- 1/2 small tomato

- 2 tablespoons of Ranch dressing

- 1-2 crisp pieces of crumbled bacon

- 1/2 hard of boiled egg (sliced in half)

- Dash pepper

- 4 ounces chopped leaf lettuce, about 2 cups

- Pinch of fresh, chopped parsley, optional

- 1/2 ounce julienned Swiss cheese

Directions:

1. Begin by grilling the chicken and then slicing it thinly.

2. Take a large plate and arrange the lettuce on it. Top this with chicken and the rest of the ingredients.

Low-Carb Fish-Based Dishes

Cheesy Tuna Casserole

Ingredients:

- 2 6-ounce of drained cans tuna

- 3 ounces fresh mushrooms (chopped)

- 1 stalk of finely chopped celery

- Xanthan gum (optional)

- 2 tablespoons of finely chopped onion

- 2 tablespoons butter

- 16 ounce bag of frozen French green beans

- 3/4 cup of heavy cream

- Salt and pepper

- 1/2 cup of chicken broth

- 4-8 ounces of shredded cheddar cheese

Directions:

1. Take a pot and cook the green beans in it, following the instructions provided on the package. Drain them well.

2. Saute the celery, mushrooms and onions in your butter until they become soft and begin to become brown.

3. Add in the broth, and then begin to boil. Give time for the liquid to reduce by half and then add in the cream. Boil again. Turn the heat down and then cook until it gets reduced and thickened, while stirring regularly to ensure that no spilling over.

4. Add in some seasonings to taste. Stir the mushroom soup mixture and tuna into the green beans mixture. Add in pepper and salt if needed. Add in the cheese and put in casserole. Bake or microwave until bubbly and hot.

Baked Salmon

Ingredients:

- 1 pound of salmon or any other fish fillet (thawed if frozen)
- Garlic powder
- Salt
- 2-4 tablespoons softened butter
- Pepper

Directions:

1. Grease some baking dish and then place the fish in it. You can choose to line it with heavy foil to make cleaning easy. Sprinkle with salt, pepper and garlic powder.

2. Use soft butter for dotting and then spread it over the surface of your fish. Bake for 6-12 minutes at 400 degrees, or until you have the thickest part of the salmon done. The amount of time to take when baking should be determined by the thickness of your fish, but be

sure that you check on a regular basis so as to avoid overcooking.

3. You can then place the fish under broiler for some minutes so that the top can be browned.

Paleo Fish Sticks

Ingredients:

- 1 ½ lbs haddock (or meaty white fish)
- about 6 oz plantain chips
- F.O.C. (fat of choice), coconut and palm can be good

Directions:

1. Crush the plantain chips in a food processor until you get the consistency of some fine bread crumbs.

2. Place the above in a bag and then add in some salt in case the chips are yet to be salted.

3. Make some strips from the fish fillets. Add few fish strips in batches and shake well until these strips get coated.

4. Take a sauce pan and melt the F.O.C in it over medium heat. Add in the coated strips and then wait for them to get brown, then turn to the other side. Each side should take not more than a minute so as to get brown. If you had cut the sticks too thick, then you should be aware that you have 4 sides to brown.

Simple Herb Crusted Salmon

Ingredients:

For Salmon

- 2 salmon fillets

- 2 tablespoons of fresh parsley

- 1 tablespoon of dijon mustard

- 1 tablespoon olive oil

- 1 heaping tablespoon of coconut flour

- salt and pepper

For Salad

- 2 cups arugula

- ¼ sliced red onion

- juice of 1 lemon

- 1 tablespoon of white wine vinegar

- 1 tablespoon of olive oil

- salt and pepper

Directions:

1. Begin by preheating the oven until it reaches 450 degrees.

2. Line a baking sheet with foil or parchment paper and then place the salmon fillets onto it.

3. Top these with salmon mustard or olive oil and then rub into the salmon.

4. Take a small bowl, and then mix parsley, salt, coconut flour and pepper in it.

5. Sprinkle the toppings onto your salmon and then pat into the salmon using your hand.

6. Transfer these into an oven for 10-15 minutes, or until you have the salmon cooked the way you need.

7. Mix your salad ingredients together as the cooking continues.

8. Place the salmon on salad and then consume.

CONCLUSION

We have come to the end of this guide. A low-carb diet is the one which restricts the amount of carbohydrates that we take. Sugars, bread and pasta are rich in carbohydrates, and these should not be part of this kind of diet. A low-carb diet is of great significance to our bodies. It can help us reduce our weight as well as reverse diabetes type 2. This is why you should know what to eat and what not to eat if you want to achieve such results.

BEFORE YOU GO

If you liked this book, would you be kind enough to give a favourable review? Every review helps!

Best Wishes,

Rose Potter

www.ingramcontent.com/pod-product-compliance
Lightning Source LLC
Chambersburg PA
CBHW071239280526
45787CB00002B/991